A MED STUDENT'S
GUIDE TO GETTING IN

(A step by step analysis of the application process
and how to develop a competitive application, from
a student's perspective)

Ernie Morton

Contents

Introduction

I remember being in your shoes a few years ago, an eager freshman in college, ready to tackle the world and become a physician. As my journey progressed and I found out more and more about what it takes to become a physician, I started to worry. The more I learned about the process, the more I realized I didn't know. It soon became apparent that I had no idea what it took to get into medical school besides getting good grades and good test scores. While those are arguably the most important factors for admission, they are far from the only factors. The medical school application consists of so much more than grades and test scores. Other areas of the application such as a personal statement, recommendation letters, and healthcare experiences are just as important.

Do not feel overwhelmed if you are in the same boat that I was. You are taking the right steps in your journey and will be just fine. By reading this book and gathering information about the application process, you are preparing for success. All of this information was once new to everyone wanting to become a physician. The information contained in this book will help you to create an exceptional plan that will result in an application to medical school.

During my own journey to medical school, I struggled to

find an accurate, succinct, and comprehensive guide to getting into medical school. I did not have time to read a 200-page book containing so much extraneous information that it was nearly impossible to process. My goal in writing this book is to provide anyone who wants to become a physician with the necessary information without all the filler. I want to help students like me, who have a true passion and desire to become a physician, to produce the best application possible. There are many things that I know now about applying to medical school that I wish I knew when I first began college. This book is the compilation of that information and all of the lessons that I have personally learned along the way.

It is my hope that this book will prepare you for the application process and put you in an even better position than I was in. Knowledge is power and the knowledge that you gain from this book will prove invaluable as you create and execute your plan for medical school admission. An understanding of the application process is essential for anyone wanting to get into medical school. So, let's begin our journey together and get you into medical school!

Part I

Chapter 1

Preface and a Fair Warning

Becoming a physician is an extremely arduous process that takes years of careful planning and immense effort in order to achieve. It is a journey that will last at least 11 years post high school (4 years of college, 4 years of medical school, and a minimum of 3 years of residency). The first thing that you need to do before progressing any further in your journey is to identify exactly why you want to become a physician and if you are pursuing this career for the right reasons. If you are wanting to become a physician for the wrong reasons, your life will be filled with countless hours of miserable working and studying. However, if becoming a physician is your true purpose in life, the journey will be well worth it and enjoyable.

There are a myriad of reasons why most people want to become a physician, but are they all the right reasons? If you want to become a doctor for the money, prestige, or because you are facing immense pressure from family, you are doing it for the wrong reasons. Believe me when I tell you that there are much easier, shorter, and quite frankly, cheaper ways to gain money and prestige. And if you are only trying to become a physician because it is what your parents want, then this is not the career for you. Putting your parent's dreams before your own is only going to lead to misery and regret. You must live your own life and choose your career for yourself. But are the "right reasons" always enough? I want to help people, I want to make the world a better place, I want to heal the sick, I am fascinated by the human body, etc. These are all common responses by young people who want to become physicians. While these are all honorable goals, it is important to notice that becoming a physician is not the only way that you can accomplish these. There are numerous other professions where you are still able to help people. There are plenty of opportunities to work for charity organizations where you can make a difference. Physician's assistants, nurses, EMTs, and many other professions help to heal those in need. Becoming a researcher is also a popular career for those who are absolutely fascinated by science. These other options are not to try and dissuade you but only to initiate deep thought on your future career and make sure that you are making the right choice for you.

I understand that it is tempting and easy to simply breeze through these paragraphs and never put any more thought into why are you doing this in the first place, but identifying why you want to become a physician is extremely important. Even if you have pondered these questions before, I challenge you to set this book aside for a moment and think about these questions:

1. Why do I want to become a physician?
2. Are these the right reasons or should I consider another profession?

Now, that you have pondered these questions and are still reading, congratulations are in order! You are headed towards many busy days and nights but also one of the most fulfilling professions in the world. Always remember your answers to the questions above. Sometimes they will be the only thing that gets you through the day. When you're up at 2am studying countless reactions for your organic chemistry final or spending all day in a lab preparing for an anatomy practical, these answers will keep you going.

There is good news regarding your journey to becoming a physician, and that news is, "once you're in, you're in". Now, I do not say this to mean that medical school is a breeze or that you can slack off because the truth is the exact opposite. It is meant to show that one of the most difficult parts of becoming a physician is admittance to medical school. Once you are admitted into a medical school, you will become a physician, as long as you continue to work hard.

However, exactly what type of physician is not guaranteed and your grades, research, board scores, and numerous other factors will determine that. (Residency application and placement is also an arduous process, but at this point in your career, you shouldn't be too worried about it.)

Even those at the bottom of their medical school class will still become physicians. They may not become the most sought-after neurosurgeon in the country, but they will still become physicians. The medical school invests large amounts of time and resources into finding the best students and once the students are there, they invest a similar amount of time and resources into keeping them there. It is extremely difficult to transfer medical schools because of the varying curriculum structures. With that being said, if a student flunks out or decides to leave a medical school, it is nearly impossible to fill that slot. Due to this fact, medical schools do their best to guarantee their students' success. They offer tutoring, employ learning specialists, and utilize numerous other tools to help you grasp the material being presented.

Chapter 2

The Application
(AMCAS and AACOMAS)

It is absolutely imperative that you have a good understanding of the application before you begin your journey. You will need to familiarize yourself with the application's systems, contents, and timeline before you apply. The application is extremely lengthy and comprehensive, thus, planning is essential to creating an application that is difficult for medical schools to turn away. Once you learn how the application process works, you can begin to plan out the next few years.

There are 2 types of medical schools in the U.S., therefore, there are 2 different application systems. The most popular and common option is MD (Medical Doctor) school which is the more traditional of the 2 options. The second option is DO (Doctor of Osteopathy) school. Osteopathy is a more recent branch of medicine that focuses on a more holistic approach to healthcare. Most of the differences between MD and DO are extremely subtle and DOs can do pretty much anything that MDs can do, and vice versa. We will go into more detail about the differences between MD and DO in 'Ch.8, Choosing a Medical School', but for now, you only need to be aware that there are 2 types of medical schools.

If you are applying to MD school, you will use the American Medical College Application Service (AMCAS), however, if you are interested in applying to DO school, then you will use the American Association of College of Osteopathic Medicine Application Service (AACOMAS). You may apply to only one type of medical school or both, it is up to you. While these 2 systems have some small differences, they ask for the same content. Once again, we'll get into more details on these differences later, but for right now it is only necessary to know the basics of the application.

The first portion of the application asks for identifying information. There is not really much to discuss here. This portion of the application will simply ask for a name, address, contact information, etc. Citizenship information is also a component and if you are not a U.S. citizen, then you may want to check either *AAMC.org* for MD school requirements or *AACOM.org* for DO requirements.

The next portion of the application deals with your academic history. In this section, you will include data on the high school you graduated from and any colleges you attended. Here is where medical schools will be able to see your GPA and any college-level courses that you have taken. You will also be asked to send in your transcripts from any colleges attended as well as to manually input your academic history into the system. To avoid any delay in the processing of your application, it is extremely important that you enter the data for your academic history exactly as it appears on your transcripts.

Discussing your experiences will make up the next portion of the application. Here, you can describe everything that you have done to prepare for the last few years. This is where you will list and describe any clubs, organizations, trips abroad, volunteer activities, research or leadership experience, job shadowing, etc. The application requires a lot of information beyond simply describing each experience. It will ask for dates, hours, and a person of contact, so make sure that you find and record all of this information while partaking in the experience. Again, we will go into much more detail in 'Ch. 4, Experiences', but we are starting with the basics (To download your free Experience log visit MasteringMedicalEducation. wordpress.com).

The next portion of your application consists of letters of recommendation. All medical schools will require letters of recommendation but they have varying standards. Some schools require letters from a physician, employer/manager, science professor, non-science professor, pre-professional advisor, committee, or other specific groups of people. The number of required letters will also vary from school to school. While some schools will only require 2 letters, others may require up to 5 letters. For information on the exact combination of letters required by each medical school, it is best to search the individual school's website or contact their admissions office. Much more detail will be given in 'Ch. 7, Letters of Recommendation'.

A personal statement is the most unique portion of the application and your chance to really show medical schools who you are. Your personal statement allows insight into who you are as a person and why you will become a great physician. The personal statement is about a page and a half to two pages in length. While a personal statement alone will not get you into medical school, a poorly written personal statement has the power to move you out of contention.

The last portion of the application contains your standardized test (MCAT) score and the schools that you have chosen to apply to. Creating an application will give you an ID number which will also be used when you take the Medical College Admissions Test (MCAT). Since you always use the same ID number, your score will automatically be synced to your application. All you will need to do is enter your test date and agree to release the results.

The final step of the application is to decide exactly which schools you wish to apply to. It is important to research medical schools to help you find the best fit for yourself. The final thing left to do is pay the application fees and then you are finished with the initial application.

Yes, that's right, there is more. The initial application is regarded as your primary application and is only the beginning of the application process. After submitting your primary application, medical schools will review it and decide whether or not to send you a secondary application. While some schools grant everyone who applies a secondary application, most schools make secondary application decisions based on a minimum set of standards determined by each individual school. For example, school X might decide to grant every student with at least a 3.00 GPA and a 495 on the MCAT a secondary application, while school Y sends everyone with a 2.80 GPA and a 498 on the MCAT a secondary application, it simply depends on the school.

So, what are these secondary applications? Secondary applications are a way for medical schools to gather other information about you that is not contained in your primary application. Schools usually gather this information through your responses to essay prompts. These essay requirements will vary in quantity, topic, and length for each individual medical school.

After you submit your secondary application, the waiting game begins. From this point, you could be waiting anywhere from a week after you submitted your secondary application to months for medical schools to contact you regarding either an interview or a decision to decline your acceptance. Almost all interviews must take place in person and on the medical school's campus, so be prepared to travel. The interview days vary but generally consist of a tour of the school, a Q&A session, and of course, the interview. There are numerous different types of interviews and the format will vary. The exact format of the interview and schedule for the interview day will differ by school.

After your interview, it is back to the waiting game. Once again, you may wait anywhere from a couple weeks to a couple of months before you hear back from the school. There are 3 decisions that the school can make. The school can grant you an acceptance, place you on their waitlist, or decline your application. Hopefully, you are granted acceptance, but if not, there is no need to fret as students are often pulled from the waitlist as late as the week before school starts. School's waitlists are also another source of variation. The length of the waitlist, average number of students taken off the waitlist each year, and whether or not the waitlist is ranked can all vary.

This is the general process for most schools, however, some schools do require more. For example, I was asked to fill out a personality assessment after one of my secondary applications. Another medical school also required a phone interview to be conducted before I was selected for an in-person interview. Overall, most schools follow the outline above but there are a few schools who require more.

So, there you have it, the application process in a nutshell. As you can see, there is a massive amount of time and energy put into the application process. It takes years of hard work to obtain the necessary skills and experience to apply to medical school. Followed by several months from primary application to acceptance. This is why it is extremely important that you do not procrastinate in any aspect of this application. It is never too early to begin obtaining any type of volunteer or healthcare experience. Do not waste your early years of college or breaks from school doing nothing. Making the most of your free time is crucial to your success. It is simply impossible to gather all of the necessary skills, experience, and knowledge required for admittance to medical school in a single year. Working hard early on will pay dividends later as you progress. Your classes only get harder and you will most likely only gain more responsibilities as you grow older, both of which will decrease the amount of time that you have to develop your application.

With all of this information, it is extremely important to stay organized. Believe me when I say that you will not be able to remember all of the information necessary to fill out the application. There will undoubtedly be portions of information that will be forgotten over the years (To download a free Experience Log visit MasteringMedicalEducation.wordpress.com). If the format of this template doesn't work for you, please feel free to design your own. The important thing is that you are keeping all of this information organized. By keeping all of this information in a single place, you will save loads of time when the moment arrives to fill out the application. You won't need to spend valuable time contacting organizations, looking up dates, nor hours. Organizational skills are crucial to surviving medical school someday, so you might as well work on developing them now.

Lastly, it will benefit you greatly to find a mentor who can help you along your journey. Everyone needs help at some point in their lives and you are no different. I know that, as a pre-med student, most things have probably come relatively easy to you but believe me when I say that this is different. The process is extremely complex and by having someone who has either gone through the process themselves or is extremely familiar with it will benefit you greatly. Don't think that your mentor has to be a doctor or a medical student. While those are great options, there are plenty of other people who are just as capable of helping you such as senior pre-med students, science faculty, or your college/university's pre-professional advisor. Becoming a physician is an extremely honorable and noble profession and you will find that there are many people out there who are willing to help you if you simply ask. Make sure to thank everyone who helps you along the way and as you progress on your journey, pay it forward and help out the next generation.

Chapter 3

Major Selection, Meeting your
Pre-Med Advisor, and Academics

Now that you have selected the right college for you, it is time to choose the proper major. A common misconception is that pre-med is a major. Pre-med is simply a term used to describe any student whose goal is to get into medical school and is taking the proper classes. For example, I was a pre-med student who majored in biomedical science and Maria was a pre-med student who majored in chemistry. As you can see, pre-med is simply a term used to group students with a similar goal (medical school) together, it is not a major. While you technically can major in any subject and be deemed as a pre-med, most students choose to major in a field of science such as biology, chemistry, physics, etc. A small portion of pre-med students choose to major in engineering, English, business, or any other field that a college offers. Although this is less common, almost every medical school class has at least 1 student with a "non-traditional" major.

Most students choose a science major as the coursework necessary to earn a degree closely aligns with required medical school pre-requisites and the material tested on the MCAT. A person majoring in chemistry will most likely take all the required courses without spending extra time in college or taking excess credits. However, a business major will most likely have to spend an extra semester or 2 beyond their own degree requirements in order to complete the necessary pre-requisites and material for the MCAT. While choosing a non-traditional major can work to differentiate you from other applicants, I would not advise it unless you are truly passionate about the subject. In the coming pages, it will be explained how choosing one of these majors makes earning a good MCAT score and science GPA even harder to achieve.

Here's a scenario for you. Let's say that we have John who is a biology major and David who is a business major. While they both spend some of their time taking the same Gen. Ed. Credits, John spends the rest of his time taking upper-level science classes and reinforcing many of the basic concepts and foundations of science. At the same time, David is spending his time taking business classes and does not use much of the basic science knowledge that he obtained through Gen. Eds. or any other science course he may have taken as an elective. Aside from the class selection, John is surrounded by other pre-med students and science faculty. John begins to build his personal network which he will use to his advantage when he applies to medical school after 4 years of college. David spends 4 years in college and is ready to graduate with his business degree, but he now has to spend an extra year taking classes full-time to satisfy medical school pre-requisites and prepare for the MCAT. David is now finally ready to apply, but his application has many weaknesses because he was unaware of all the things he should have done during college to prepare to apply.

The point of this scenario is not to dissuade you from choosing a major outside of the science field. My hope is to simply make you aware of the extra challenges that arise from being a non-traditional major. If you decide to choose a major outside of science, it is important that you use your elective credits to take science classes. These will not only expand your knowledge base but they will keep your scientific knowledge current and fresh. Thus, helping to reduce the amount of time necessary to finish pre-reqs and prepare for the MCAT. Secondly, it is important to partake in activities and experiences that you can use on your application while you are completing your degree. There is no way that you will be able to create a competitive application if you wait until you're done with your other major to begin gaining the necessary experience to apply. Science majors will have dedicated 3 years to gaining this experience and there simply is not enough time for you to gain a similar amount.

The great news about selecting a major is that this is not a choice that you will need to make by yourself. At college, you are surrounded by countless faculty and staff that are there to help you achieve your dream. I would advise for you to speak with the college's pre-medical advisor as soon as possible. Discussing major options is a great excuse to meet your pre-med advisor and develop a working relationship. The pre-med advisor should be able to help answer any questions that you have regarding medical school and point you in the direction that is best for you. They will be able to give you information on not only what the popular major choices for pre-med students are, but a whole plethora of other information such as clubs to join, activities to participate in, professors and courses to take, and every other aspect of having a successful pre-medical college career.

The pre-med advisor is going to play a large part in the next few years of your life as you prepare for medical school. As we progress through this book, the pre-med advisor will be brought up time and time again. By the conclusion of this book, you will grasp exactly how crucial a good relationship with your pre-med advisor is and how beneficial they can be. It is best to get to know them as early as possible so that you can receive the greatest amount of help. They can be a great resource and many medical students credit much of their success in undergrad to the help and guidance of their pre-med advisor.

Although most schools will give you until the end of your second year to officially declare a major, I would advise that you do it as soon as possible. Obviously, take your time and do not rush to declare a major, but the sooner you declare a major, the sooner you may begin to plan out your classes. If you wait too long to declare a major, then you run the risk of taking classes that will not count towards graduation and could possibly be a waste of time and money. Once you have declared a major, I would advise for you to create a 4-year plan depicting each semester and exactly which courses you will take each semester. While this plan does not have to be set in stone, it will help when attempting to plan out other future events such as preparing for and taking the MCAT and applying to medical school. Feel free to readjust your plan as you progress in your journey, but creating, modifying, and executing a plan are essential skills to develop in life (To download your free 4-year plan visit MasteringMedicalEducation.wordpress.com)

There are certain pre-reqs that you need to have completed before taking the MCAT and applying to medical school. By writing out your plan, you can make sure that you have all of the requirements met in time. Make sure that you include at least 1 sociology, psychology, and biochemistry course in your 4-year plan. (Taking introductory courses in these subjects should be sufficient.) These subjects are being required by more and more medical schools every year and they make up a large portion of the MCAT, so you need to take them. Even if they are not explicitly needed for your major, they will usually cover some sort of Gen. Ed. Credit and will count towards graduation.

Once you have completed your 4-year plan, you should take it to your pre-med advisor where they can go over it with you to make sure that the order of classes is correct and the courses necessary to take the MCAT and apply to medical school are completed in time. Once again, this is another great opportunity to work with your pre-med advisor and become more comfortable with them. Please do not be afraid to make mistakes or be nervous about meeting with your pre-med advisor. Developing a 4-year plan for your courses is more challenging than most people think and if you've made a few mistakes, it is okay. That is what your advisor is there for. They would love to help you create a successful plan and would more than likely be thrilled by your initiative for creating a plan.

As mentioned above, it is also important to plan when you want to take the MCAT and begin applying to medical school. The most common timeline has students taking the MCAT and submitting their applications during the summer between their junior and senior year of college. In this timeline, the student will spend their senior year completing secondary applications, attending interviews, and preparing to begin medical school a few months after graduation. A common alternative to this is to wait until after you graduate to take the MCAT, and doing so will allow you to have what we call a "gap year", which is simply a year where you are not enrolled in school anywhere. This gap year will allow you to dedicate all of your time to the MCAT and application as well as provide you extra time to gain experience that you can use to strengthen your application. There is no penalty for taking a gap year as long as you are being productive. A gap year is not a time to slack off and do nothing. Medical schools want to see that you use your time productively and a gap year is no different. Even if you decide that you would like to take a gap year to decompress, strengthen your application, or anything else from a long list of reasons, make sure that it is a productive use of time and that you can articulate that. Do not simply take a gap year and do nothing but travel and kick back. Taking a gap year for purposes of vacation or other similar activities is not viewed very favorably by medical school admissions committees.

You may notice that there is no chart for the summer semesters on the 4-year plan (visit MasteringMedicalEducation.wordpress.com to download). Instead, there are empty bullet points. These should be used to list activities or experiences that you hope to partake in during the summer, i.e. taking the MCAT or applying to medical school. I feel that summer vacations are a great time for you to do something other than school. You are simply too busy during the school year to participate in some things and this time away provides a great chance for you to become more involved. Whether this means more time spent volunteering at the hospital, taking an EMT course, or participating in a summer research program, there are many great opportunities available in the summer that allow you to make the most of your time away from school. However, perhaps you took a while to decide on pre-med and are somewhat behind, so you decide to use the summer to catch up by a course or two. This may be what is best for you personally. If you choose to do this, make sure that you are still partaking in other activities as well so that other applicants do not get even further ahead of you. Everyone will be different and there is no perfect way to get into medical school, but I truly feel that summers should be spent doing something besides school that increases your chances of earning an acceptance.

Now that we have discussed selecting the best major for yourself, it is time to talk about what exactly medical schools are expecting from you in terms of course selection and GPA. You do not need a 4.0 to get into medical school, but the higher your GPA and more challenging your schedule, the better. No matter what anyone else tells you, GPA and MCAT scores are the most important parts of the primary application. Earning a great GPA and MCAT should always be your first priority. Do not do anything that will negatively affect your GPA or MCAT score. Do not partake in hours of research, volunteering, and work to beef up your application if you have no time to study and your GPA suffers. Obtaining a good GPA and MCAT score are your best weapons when it comes to being granted an interview. As a pre-medical student, you are most likely already a high achiever and don't need to be prodded to always give your best, but remember, while your GPA does not have to be perfect, it still has to be above average.

When it comes to GPA, there are going to be 2 things that medical schools look at. The first of which is your normal or traditional GPA. This is the GPA that your school provides you with on transcripts. The second is your science GPA. This is separate from your normal GPA and is calculated in the same manner as a normal GPA, except it only includes data from biology, chemistry, physics, and math classes. A science GPA helps medical schools when comparing applicants by reducing variations in course schedules. Your science GPA is generally considered more important and will be weighed more heavily than your normal GPA as it is a better comparison tool. As mentioned before, it is best to aim as high as possible but if you can achieve a normal GPA of 3.8 and a science GPA of 3.65, then by the time you are ready to apply, you should be in good shape. For those of you who are unfamiliar with how to calculate a GPA, an A – is a 3.7 so you will need to average nearly an A – in all of your science classes to be where we would like. Also, these are general goals to help you get you into a medical school but GPA information will vary for each medical school. If you have a specific medical school in mind or there is only 1 medical school in your state or region, it is best to go on their website and locate this information before you set any goals concerning GPA.

What about Advanced Placement (AP) and College Level Examination Program (CLEP) credits? Pre-med students often ask how medical schools view AP and CLEP credits and how these types of credits affect your GPA calculation. In general, medical schools accept credits that were granted to you due to your performance on an AP or CLEP exam. While it is nice to receive free credits and not have to take a course, perhaps for the second time, there is also a downside to consider. While medical schools will give you credit for these classes, they will not assign a grade for them. Thus, your science GPA will be calculated with fewer credits. Let's say that by the time you are ready to apply to medical school you have completed 50 credits of science classes. Of these 50 credits, 8 of them are AP credits for biology and chemistry. So, while the medical school will grant you credit for biology and chemistry, they will not factor them into your science GPA. This will cause your science GPA to be calculated using only 42 credits, not 50. This decrease in credits will cause every other class to be weighted more heavily and have a greater effect on your science GPA. Also, since you passed the AP test, it is safe to say that if you retook the course, you most likely would have received an A or A-. This would most likely boost your science GPA and counteract a subpar grade in a more challenging course later on. Keep in mind that the more AP and CLEP credits you have, the greater this effect. Overall, it makes sense to accept any AP or CLEP credit that you earn but do be aware of the effect that it can have on your science GPA.

If you are concerned that your GPAs are too low, do not fret too much. While GPA is one of the most important areas on your application, there are ways to compensate for having a GPA in the lower range of applicants. The simplest way to make up for a lower GPA is to earn an amazing MCAT score. Therefore, if your GPA is not where you would like it and there is no time to bring it up, I would advise that you put an extreme amount of effort into the MCAT. Medical schools understand that sometimes circumstances arise that will cause an applicant to have less than desired performance in a course or throughout a semester. The MCAT is an opportunity to demonstrate that you might not have received a good grade in the course but still understand the material. A second option is to retake some of the courses that you performed poorly in. However, I would only advise this if you didn't do well in the course. So, while your university will most likely replace the grade on your transcripts, medical schools will use the average of the 2 grades. Due to the averaging of grades by medical schools, you must get an A in the class that you are retaking or else it is not worth the time and effort. If you earned a B in a class the first time and then retake the class and earn an A− the second time, medical schools will consider you earned a B+ in the class. In my mind, this is too large of an investment of time and money for such a small return. As far as medical schools are concerned, you have only increased your grade for the course by a half a letter grade. This is simply not worth it and I think this time and money would be better spent preparing for the MCAT to make up for a sub-par GPA. If, however, you earned a C initially and an A the second time around, medical schools will consider this a B, so you have increased your grade by a full letter grade. Improvements in grades of this size are worth the investment.

Your course selection is more important than most people think and plays an integral part in your GPA. Choosing the correct courses is a balancing act between creating a challenging enough schedule that medical schools are satisfied but not so challenging that your GPA suffers. The first thing to consider when selecting courses is what courses are required for admittance into medical schools. While technically medical schools only require 1 year of biology, physics, English, and 2 years of chemistry (through organic chemistry), these are only minimum requirements. Most medical schools will have additional requirements beyond these but they vary from school to school. It is best to check the required pre-requisites for some medical schools that interest you in order to gain a better understanding of exactly what you will need.

There are a few courses that may or may not be required by a medical school that you still need to take. These courses are introductory psychology, introductory sociology, and bio-chemistry. You need to take these courses as they are all tested on the MCAT and make up a large portion of the exam. There are also a few more courses that are not required by medical schools or directly tested on the MCAT but are highly recommended. These courses are genetics, statistics, anatomy and physiology, pathophysiology, immunology, epidemiology, and medical ethics. Since these subjects are all taught in medical school, they are not as imperative as the previous 3. However, having a good understanding of them prior to beginning medical school will benefit you greatly. Your previous experience with these subjects will allow you a small mental break or some time to destress while you go over the material for a second time in medical school.

Depending on your major, it can be somewhat difficult to fit all of these courses into your schedule in time. If you are a science major, then most likely your program will already require many of these courses but it is still important to double check. If you are a non-science major, then fitting these classes in can be a lot trickier and may require taking a course or two over the summer as well as spending time at a university after you have successfully completed your degree's requirements. This is why is it important to design a 4-year plan, or maybe a 5-year plan if you are a non-science major, and go over it with your pre-med advisor. Proper preparation will help to ensure that everything runs smoothly and that you stay on track during your journey.

In summary, academics make up a significant portion of your application and they are one of, if not the most, important areas for medical school admission. A strong academic performance is imperative to earning a spot in medical school. It is essential that you take a proactive approach when considering your GPA and course selection. Choosing a major early on will allow you to design a 4 or 5-year plan that consists of all the required classes completed in a timely manner and gives you an opportunity to meet your pre-med advisor. Although it is recommended that you choose a science major, this is not required. While a non-traditional major does pose unique challenges, if there is something outside of science that you are passionate about, then go for it.

Remember to always do your best and shoot for a 4.0 but if you struggle with a few courses, you will still be okay. There are other ways to make up for a low grade or GPA but it is much easier to do to earn the necessary grade the first time. Also, do not forget that your science classes are weighted more heavily by medical schools and should take precedence over other classes. GPA, more specifically science GPA, and MCAT scores are the 2 most important factors for receiving an interview invitation. Do not take on so much that your GPA begins to suffer, it is extremely important. Academics are key to medical school acceptance and should be treated as such.

Chapter 4

Experiences

So, what else do you need besides a high GPA and MCAT score to get into medical school? In short, you will need experience. Exactly how much and what type of experience will vary from person to person. There are so many options when it comes to choosing experiences during your undergrad and each one has its own pros and cons. This can make choosing the best experiences for yourself extremely challenging, but do not worry. We will take a detailed look at the experiences section of the application, discuss what medical schools are looking for, and provide information on many popular options for pre-med students. This chapter separates experiences into 3 categories: healthcare experiences, research experiences, and volunteer experiences. Preferably, you will devote some time to all 3 areas. However, you do not need to split your time equally between them and if you are truly passionate about a certain area then it is acceptable for it to take up more of your time.

Before we get any further into specific experiences or medical school's expectations, let's take a look at the experience section of the application in more detail. Although we have not yet gone into great detail on MD vs DO, you should remember that there are 2 application systems. The system that you use is determined by the type of medical school you are applying to, MD schools use AMCAS and DO schools use AACOMAS. There are some differences which we will note, but for the most part, they are the same.

Both application systems have an experiences section that will allow you to list and describe up to 15 experiences that you participated in during your undergraduate career. Aside from providing a general description of the experience, you will need to enter information regarding dates, times, and a contact person. Considering that you will apply later on in your journey and some of these experiences will have taken place a few years ago, it is best to gather all of this information while you are participating in the experience. I have created an experience log which you can download for free by visiting MasteringMedicalEducation.wordpress.com. Obtaining, recording, and keeping track of this information can save you loads of time and stress when it comes to filling out the application. Trying to track down all of this information years later can be extremely difficult and sometimes unsuccessful. While medical schools don't always reach out to your person of contact, you do not want to take the risk of providing false information which will almost certainly lead to a denial.

While both the AMCAS and AACOMAS experience sections are very similar, there are some differences. The AMCAS will allow you up to 700 characters to describe each experience as well as identify up to 3 of your experiences as being the most meaningful. Selecting one of your experiences as most meaningful will allow you an additional 1325 characters to describe this experience in more detail as well as explain why the experience is so important to you. The AACOMAS is somewhat different in that you are given only 600 characters to describe your experiences and none can be selected as most meaningful. However, the AACOMAS has additional achievements and continuing education courses sections. The awards section allows you to list any awards that you have earned during your undergraduate years. The continuing education courses section allows you to upload a certificate for any extra courses that you may have taken. An Emergency Medical Technician (EMT) or Certified Nurse Assistant or Aide (CNA) course are examples of courses that could be listed here. By listing experiences in one of these additional sections, you will free up space in the experiences section, thus allowing you to discuss more experiences than on your AMCAS application.

In general, medical schools like to see a breadth of experiences as well as the longevity of certain experiences. This means that medical schools like to see that you have done a lot of different things during your college career but they also like to see a commitment to the things that you are most passionate about. If you are trying new things and discover that there is something that you have an interest in or a passion for, then by all means stick with it. Medical schools love to see you progress over the years from perhaps a general member of a club to eventually taking on more responsibility. For example, if after 4 years in an organization you're still only a general member, it is not as impressive to a medical school as a person who after 4 years is in one of the leadership positions.

While partaking in experiences is important, it is also necessary to gain some leadership experience. As a future physician, you will often lead a team of medical professionals and developing these organizational and leadership skills during your undergraduate years is looked upon very favorably. While you do not have to become the president or other high-ranking member of every organization that you are a part of, it will greatly behoove you to have advanced into a leadership role in some way, shape, or form.

Working your way up to a leadership role can take some time and that is why I would advise you to begin gaining experience as soon as possible. Not only so that you have the time to work your way up, but more importantly so that you can find something that you have enough interest in to become more involved. Most likely, you will not love everything that you try and it could take some time to find something that you enjoy. Do not take a leadership role in an organization simply for the sake of gaining leadership experience. It will be extremely challenging to be a good leader if you are in charge of something that you do not enjoy or find worthwhile. Instead, place your time and energy into finding the right opportunity for you and pursuing it wholeheartedly.

As with everything else in this book, DO NOT PROCRAS-TINATE. Many students feel that they have 3 or 4 years to gain experience and they put off participating in clubs, volunteering, research, etc. until later in their college careers. This is the wrong approach and will only lead to unnecessary work and stress further down the road. The earlier you begin gaining experience, the better but make sure to not overdo it. As mentioned in the previous chapter, your GPA is extremely important and you do not want to do so much that your GPA suffers. I would advise participating in no more than 2 weekly obligations during your first semester in college or until you are adapted to college and the rigors that are associated with it.

So, let's begin with the first category, healthcare experiences. These experiences will become some of the most defining moments of your undergraduate career. They will most likely further solidify your desire to become a physician and possibly steer you towards a specific area of medicine. While there are a myriad of options for healthcare experiences, we will discuss a few of the most popular options. The following are not the only ways to gain healthcare experience and please feel free to pursue other options outside of those discussed. These are mentioned to make you aware of what many other pre-med students are doing and to give you ideas of similar activities that you can partake in.

Job shadowing is a very popular way to gain healthcare experience. In general, this consists of following a physician for a period of time and observing their day to day routine and activities. This could range from scrubbing in and observing a knee replacement surgery to observing a physician as they evaluate patients at their clinic. If you have a specific area of medicine that interests you, it is best to shadow that specific type of physician. However, shadowing a physician of another specialty could also expose you to a side of medicine that you are not as familiar with. Both situations have their benefits and, overall, it is better to have some shadowing experience than none. Shadowing a physician is also a great opportunity to get to know a physician on a personal level. This can often lead to receiving advice and opinions on medical school and possibly even a letter of recommendation later on if everything goes well. While shadowing is a great experience, it can be hard to partake in due to Health Insurance Portability and Accountability Act (HIPPA) laws and a lack of willing doctors. I would always advise asking any physician you come in contact with if they are willing to let you shadow them, but do not be discouraged if they say no. Patient privacy and HIPPA are very complex issues and perhaps a physician is not allowed to have pre-med students shadow them. Whatever the reason though, it never hurts to ask.

Taking a medical mission trip abroad is also a very popular option among pre-med students. A group of students will usually gather donations of vital supplies and then travel to a less developed or a less prosperous country and provide care to the local population. The group of students are usually accompanied by physicians from the U.S. or they will team up with a group of local physicians when they arrive. Either way, the students will assist the medical staff in all types of care. These trips are often considered life-changing by the students who go and usually provide a wealth of information to use when constructing your personal statement. While these trips are amazing, they are often extremely expensive. Most organizations provide ways to help students fundraise, but students often end up paying a significant portion out of pocket. These trips are extremely popular and many pre-med students do participate in them but they are not a necessity for medical school admission. They are valued by medical schools the same as a healthcare experience in the states. There is no difference in a medical school's view of volunteering at a hospital in the U.S. versus volunteering at a hospital in a third world country. Just because you traveled thousands of miles to volunteer does not mean that it is valued any greater. All in all, these are great experiences and if you have the opportunity and funds to partake in one, I would highly recommend it. On a personal note, I was able to go on 2 of these trips and I found them both to be life-changing and priceless experiences. Nevertheless, if you are unable to participate for any reason, do not feel as though you are going to be disadvantaged when it comes to applying.

While job shadowing and a trip abroad are usually singular experiences, there are also activities that you can partake in on a weekly basis to gain healthcare experience. Joining a club or organization is a great way to gain healthcare experience on a regular basis and usually provides opportunities for leadership roles in the future. There are numerous clubs and organizations for pre-med students at every college and I would advise that you explore a few different ones before deciding to join.

Most colleges have a pre-medical club, pre-health professions club, or a similar club. These clubs usually feature speakers such as medical school admission's reps, physicians, or college advisors. These featured speakers will come and discuss certain topics, all geared towards gaining acceptance into medical school. Most of these clubs are geared towards educating and assisting pre-med students on the application process and what it entails. Another popular club is Beta Beta

Beta (TriBeta). TriBeta is a national biology fraternity and most larger schools will have a chapter. This is not your stereotypical fraternity with a frat house and crazy parties like you see in the movies. TriBeta is an academic fraternity for both men and women who are interested in biology. While TriBeta is not geared specifically towards medical school admission, it is still a great organization that provides many of the same experiences and opportunities as the previous options. Yet another similar type of organization is the Minority Association of Pre-Med Students (MAPS). While this organization is geared towards minority students, anyone and everyone is welcome to join. MAPS is a nationwide organization and like TriBeta, most larger schools will have a chapter. Please do not feel as though you must join one of these organizations. They are simply popular suggestions and should serve as a guide for what you are looking for in an organization.

While these are all great organizations to be a part of and will help you to gain healthcare experience, they are not going to help pay your bills. If you need to work during college, there are several jobs that will help you to gain valuable healthcare experience as well as provide a steady paycheck. These jobs are very popular among pre-medical students and the great news is that some of them require little to no training to apply.

Becoming a medical scribe can help you gain first-hand insight into a physician's routine with little to no training required to apply. As a scribe, your job is relatively simple and straightforward. You will follow a physician and record everything that happens into medical records or documents. This is a great job that will allow you to directly observe a physician while getting paid. There is no special training needed to apply but there will be some training required once you are hired to become familiar with specific documents and learn some shorthand terms, i.e. HTN stands for hypertension. Overall, this job is not incredibly difficult and provides a great opportunity to observe and assist physicians at work.

While becoming a scribe is a great opportunity to gain healthcare experience, it is not very hands-on. If you would prefer something where you are physically interacting with an individual, then becoming a phlebotomist is a great option. This is the practice of drawing blood from an individual for testing or other medical purposes. While this job does require some skills, in most states you can usually apply with no formal training and learn on the job. There are a number of different places that you can work as a phlebotomist but plasma donation centers, blood donation centers, and medical diagnostic laboratories are the most common. Please remember that this job will require you to insert a needle into an individual. If this is something that you are not comfortable with or you are deathly afraid of needles, you may want to consider another job.

While the previous jobs require no formal training or certifications, they do not let you provide much, if any, care to individuals. There are jobs that are even more hands-on than phlebotomy and also allow you to provide varying levels of basic care to individuals. Becoming a certified nursing assistant or aide (CNA) or an emergency medical technician (EMT) are both great jobs that allow you to provide care to individuals. While the thought of actually providing care to patients is very enticing, there is a small downside. Both jobs require that you invest a significant amount of time and effort into a class before having to pass some sort of licensing exam to earn your certification.

A CNA will provide basic levels of care to individuals, usually under the supervision of a registered nurse. As a CNA, you will assist individuals with activities of daily living such as toileting, ambulating, transferring, or bathing, just to name a few. On occasion, you will also be asked to obtain vitals or provide basic first aid. The exact type of care provided to individuals will vary slightly based on the environment that you choose to work in. Working at a long-term care facility will differ slightly from working at a hospital. The differences between the 2 should be considered when looking for a job. For example, working in a hospital is probably going to be more stressful than a long-term care facility. However, working in a hospital will expose you to more aspects of medicine and healthcare than working at a long-term care facility. Additionally, patients in a hospital are, for the most part, temporary, while residents of a long-term facility are there for a long period of time. If you value long-term relationships with the people that you are caring for, then it would be better to work at a long-term care facility. Both are great environments to work and learn in as a CNA, yet they each have their own unique pros and cons that you should consider before looking for a job. Also, these are not the only workplace options for CNAs, these are simply the most popular.

The downside to becoming a CNA is the amount of training and the cost that is required to obtain your certification. There are some facilities that will hire you without a license and pay for your training and certification, but these are few and far between for students. Most organizations are only willing to do this for employees who are going to be working full-time and plan to stay with the organization for multiple years. Most students need to take the course before they will be hired. In general, obtaining a CNA license requires taking a class that requires between 80 and 100 hours of coursework and can last anywhere from 2 weeks to 2 months. During a CNA course, you will spend roughly a third of the time in the classroom, a third in the skills laboratory, and a third at a long-term care facility. Finding the time to dedicate to the class and testing can be difficult but summer or winter breaks are a perfect opportunity.

Aside from the time commitment, cost is also a drawback of becoming a CNA. These classes are relatively expensive and usually cost at least $1,000. After you have successfully completed the class, you will receive a certificate that will allow you to attempt a state licensing exam. These state exams often consist of both a written portion and skills assessment. After you pass the state exam, you will be eligible to receive your certification. The state exam and receiving your certification also have costs associated with them which will total a few hundred dollars. The rules and regulations vary by state and this is just a general outline, but as you can see, there is a decent investment needed to become a CNA.

While this job is not glamorous by any means, it is a great way to develop your interpersonal abilities and actually provide care to individuals. Being a CNA can be a truly gratifying experience which will help you develop many of the intangibles that are needed to become a great physician. If this is something that you are interested in, I would advise that you look into the requirements for your particular state and fit it into your 4-year plan.

Working as an emergency medical technician (EMT) is another great option for pre-med students, especially those who have an interest in emergency medicine. As an EMT, you will respond to emergency calls, deliver immediate care to the injured or ill, and transport to the appropriate medical facility if necessary. You will be administering medical care in a highly stressful environment which is as close to a practicing physician as possible. The unique situations that you will experience as an EMT will serve you extremely well as you become a physician. Becoming an EMT will allow you an opportunity to provide a high level of care to individuals and possibly even save a life.

As an EMT, you will respond to numerous different incidents such as car accidents, dog bites, heart attacks, strokes, and any other unplanned medical emergency. You will most likely be the first medical personnel on the scene and it will be your job to manage the patient using the skills that you have learned. EMTs are expected to be proficient in CPR, AED use, oxygen use, stabilizing head and neck injuries, etc. For those of you looking for a more intense challenge and chance to save a life, then EMT is a great option for you.

Nonetheless, there are drawbacks and challenges to working as an EMT. The first of which is the length of time that it takes to receive your EMT certification. Most EMT courses are taught at community colleges and take place over the course of an entire semester. There are more intense programs that you can complete in as little as 3 weeks but these are not as readily available. Aside from the huge time commitment, these courses can also be very expensive and cost upwards of $2000. After you have completed a skills exam and worked approximately 48 hours, then you will be eligible to take a national certification exam. As you can see, it takes quite a lot of time and effort to become an EMT. Another challenge with becoming an EMT is the hours of work. Most EMT shifts vary from 8 to 24 hours and change from week to week. It can be challenging to find the time in your busy schedule as well as make the rotating shifts fit within your class schedule. Twenty-four-hour shifts can also disrupt your normal sleeping routine which can lead to issues with your academics and, as stated before, your GPA is your number 1 priority.

Overall, becoming an EMT is a great option for pre-med students who work well in stressful situations and want to provide lifesaving care. If you are interested in working as an EMT, I would highly encourage it. However, make sure that you have enough time to complete the necessary requirements and work as an EMT. Medical schools may not look very favorably upon earning a certification and never putting your skills to use.

All of the healthcare experiences that we covered are great options for a pre-med student to build up their application. While you do not need to experience every option we discussed, I would advise that you try out as many as you can. It is just as important to find out what you do not enjoy as it is to discover the areas that you are most passionate about.

Experience as much as you can and stick with the ones that interest you the most. Healthcare experience is an important component of your application and beyond. These experiences will begin to shape you as a future physician and most likely contribute to many of your responses to secondary essays and interview questions.

Now that we have discussed a number of great healthcare experiences, it is time to get into our second type of experience, which is research. While research is not a requirement for most medical schools, it is looked upon very favorably. Of all the experiences needed for medical school admittance, research is probably the most important. It shows medical schools that you have spent time developing a scientific mind and are capable of working with ideas that are on the edges of current knowledge. Medical schools often conduct large amounts of research and love to have their students involved as much as possible. Participating in research as an undergraduate indicates to medical schools that you will most likely be willing to participate in research at their institution as well. While research is not required for admittance, I would highly recommend it.

Even if research is something that does not interest you at the moment, I would urge that you give it a chance before completely writing it off. If your enthusiasm towards research is truly lacking then there are a couple of things that you can do to make the experience more enjoyable. You should try to find a research topic that interests you or speak with your favorite professor to inquire about joining their research team. Having a genuine interest in the topic and working with people who you enjoy will go a long way in making the project more enjoyable. It is okay if you are interested in a research topic that does not pertain to medicine. While most medical schools would prefer that you were a part of medical research, any research experience is better than none. Nevertheless, if you choose to participate in research that does not relate to medicine, make sure that you are able to discuss how your experience within another field will help to make you a better physician in the future.

Although the focus of this book is gaining admittance to medical school, I would like to mention that research is most likely something that you are going to have to do in medical school. While applying for residency, you will be competing with many other talented individuals and research is a great way to differentiate yourself. If you are interested in a relatively competitive medical specialty (dermatology, plastic surgery, otolaryngology, neurosurgery or pretty much any type of surgery) or a highly coveted residency program in another specialty, then research is practically a must. Everyone applying for these residencies is going to have great academics and board scores, thus you will need something more to separate you from the crowd. If you are considering a specialty that is not as competitive (family medicine, internal medicine, pediatrics), then there may be no need to do research as residencies in these fields are not as hard to obtain. Regardless of what specialty you are considering, participating in research during medical school is only going to help you become a better physician and scientist in the future. Most medical students will end up participating in research during medical school, thus it is beneficial to begin developing your skillset as soon as possible.

Even for those who are extremely interested in participating in research, it can be a challenge to find research opportunities. And once you have found opportunities, it can be even more challenging to become a part of them. While there is often quite a bit of research happening at universities, the opportunities for participation can be hard to locate, limited in number, and competitive to join.

Most universities or organizations will have a research page or tab on their main website. This page will contain information on all current research projects and some will even allow you to filter the research projects by topic, department, faculty involved, etc. Whatever the case, I would advise you to look through the webpage to locate projects that are of interest to you. At this point, you should reach out to faculty and inquire about joining their research project. While I would advise scheduling a face to face meeting, this can often be difficult due to both you and the professors' hectic schedules. If a face to face meeting is not possible then a simple email inquiry will suffice, but I have found face to face meetings to produce better results.

During meetings or email correspondence, it is important that you are professional and courteous. Conducting yourself professionally will go a long way when trying to develop a working relationship with a faculty member. Also, make sure that you are familiar with the faculty's research. Do not simply send a generic email to 30 professors and expect to get a response. You are going to have to spend some time becoming familiar with each faculty member's research. You by no means need to be an expert on the topic but you must know enough to understand the basis of the research and be able to ask educated questions on the topic. This research will help you to show interest when composing an email to the professor by referencing their current work. Showing some interest in the faculty's research will help to set you apart from other students hoping to join their research project. The final piece of communicating with faculty is to have a resume or Curriculum Vitae (CV) ready, and it wouldn't hurt to also include a copy of your current academic record. A resume, CV, and academic record will all serve as support for your cause. You can talk all you want, but without the necessary supporting material, your words will hold little weight. Developing a resume takes time and effort. Even if there is not much on your resume, do not be embarrassed or not try to become involved. Most faculty understand that everyone must start somewhere and you will eventually find someone who is willing to give you a chance. Please do not get discouraged if faculty do not respond or turn down your offer. Persistence is key and believe me when I say that, eventually, you will be accepted to a project if you follow these steps.

Another source of research opportunities are your current and past professors. Hopefully you have developed a relationship with your professors as this can be a huge benefit when asking to join their research team. If a professor has witnessed your intelligence, work ethic, or any other positive trait during their class and/or office hours, they are more likely to accept your offer. Do not be afraid to reach out to your professors regarding their research. Most professors have a true passion for the topic that they are investigating and would love to discuss it with you. Similar to emailing professors, make sure that you are prepared and have gained some basic knowledge on the topic. While inquiring about the topic and project, make sure that it is a good fit for you before asking to join on. Once again, do not get discouraged if a professor turns you away. There are only a limited number of spots available for undergraduates and it is not uncommon for these spots to be filled before a research project even begins.

Yet another potential source of research opportunities is your pre-med advisor. While they are most likely not conducting any research, they have plenty of experience connecting students with research opportunities. Your advisor should be able to point you in the right direction or introduce you to the right people. Their recommendation will often go a long way towards helping you to gain a research position. Beyond the research taking place at your university, your pre-med advisor may also have knowledge regarding summer research opportunities.

During the summer months, many universities and private labs or research companies will hire students to help with some of their projects. For those of you who do not particularly like research, this can be a great way to gain some research experience in a short amount of time without committing to a project for 1 to 2 years. The downside, however, to these summer research programs is that you are less likely to become published as you will most likely depart before the project is finished. Aside from their short duration, there is another benefit to many of these programs. They usually provide pay or a stipend and take place all over the country. Some students apply to programs that are far from home and, if accepted, they have the opportunity to experience another part of the country as well as build up their resume.

As future physicians, most of us are passionate about giving back and volunteering is a great way to demonstrate to medical schools your desire to make a difference. There is a plethora of volunteering opportunities, both in and out of healthcare. These experiences can often be intermingled with healthcare and research experience or they can stand alone. Regardless of how we classify our experiences, it is important that we discuss volunteering and its relevance in creating the best possible application.

Before you begin volunteering, it is important that you understand what medical schools are looking for in terms of volunteering. Similar to joining clubs and other organizations, medical schools like to see both a variety of volunteer experiences as well as continued dedication to a particular cause. Even though there is no requirement concerning how many hours you need to spend a year volunteering or how you gather those hours, you need to volunteer. In general, I would advise that you volunteer at least 50 hours a year and this should be the absolute minimum. While this may sound like quite a bit, it is less than an hour a week over the course of the year. How you earn these hours is totally up to you as they can be earned during a healthcare experience or at a completely separate event. Even though you may choose to earn these hours however you want, I would advise that you do not volunteer for more than 3 to 4 different causes a year. This shows little commitment to any particular cause and medical schools would prefer to see you volunteer a few hours a week for the same cause over the course of a semester or school year. This does not mean that you cannot volunteer for a singular event, but you should try to limit those experiences. Obviously, there are many great singular events that you can and should volunteer for such as disaster relief efforts or Relay for Life events, but they come at a cost. If you are interested in some of these events then by all means volunteer, but I would make sure to limit them. Keep in mind that you will need to list and describe your experiences on your application. There are only 15 spots to list all of your experiences gained during your undergraduate years (healthcare, research, and volunteer) and if you volunteer at too many different events, you will simply not be able to list them all. If an experience is not contained in your application, then as far as the medical school is concerned, it didn't happen and you can gain no benefit from an event that is not contained in your application.

While it is nice to volunteer in a healthcare setting, it is also beneficial to garner other real-world experiences outside of medicine. While a majority of your time spent volunteering should be in a healthcare field, it is completely okay to spend large amounts of time elsewhere. Some pre-med students have a passion for animals and spend large amounts of time volunteering at the local animal shelter. Other pre-med students have a passion for helping the homeless or the hungry and will spend most of their time volunteering at the local soup kitchen or food pantry. Whatever the cause, it's important that you volunteer outside of medicine to become a more well-rounded applicant. Medical schools want their classes to be composed of unique individuals who can all learn from and teach one another. Gaining different experiences outside of medicine is a great way to help differentiate yourself. Everyone will have similar experiences of volunteering in a healthcare setting, so this is really a chance to make yourself unique. Find a cause outside of healthcare that you are passionate about and spend time giving back. As with any experience that you partake in, keep in mind how this will make you a better physician in the future. If you are unable to relate an experience to being a physician in some way, then it is probably best to choose another option. A few examples of locations or organizations that you can volunteer at outside of healthcare are a local food pantry, animal shelter, homeless shelter, elementary schools, Habitat for Humanity, the Red Cross, and United Way.

Most pre-med students will have similar volunteer experiences in healthcare as there is only so much that a student with little to no medical training can actually partake in. To make things even more challenging, HIPAA regulations and policy further impede access for pre-med students. Despite the difficulties, there are still a decent number of volunteer experiences available in the healthcare field. Hospitals, long-term care facilities, and blood drives are all popular options for volunteering. (Medical volunteer trips abroad also fall into this category but those were already discussed in more detail earlier.) The tasks and responsibilities will vary from location to location, but, overall, you will be tasked with assisting with some of the basic responsibilities of the facility such as laundry, restocking supplies, delivering food, cleaning, etc. While it is important to gather time volunteering in a healthcare facility, make sure that it is not a waste of your time. If you are volunteering at a hospital and all you are doing is changing dirty linens, then you are probably not learning too much. There is not much worth in saying that you volunteered in a hospital if you only changed sheets. Make sure that you are actually gaining insight and knowledge from the experience. If this is not the case, then I would advise that you conclude volunteering there and find something more productive to do with your time.

Now, I understand that we have discussed a lot of

information and it may seem overwhelming, but please relax. While choosing what experiences to participate in and when to participate can seem complex, it is not as hard as you may think. Simply try many different things then stick with the experiences that you enjoy and dump the experiences that are a drag. You will get the most out of participating in experiences that you truly enjoy. There is no secret formula to experiences and exactly what you participate in and to what level will vary from person to person. Remember that while It is not a must to divide your time equally between all 3 categories, you need to have some experience in each category. Also, protect your GPA, do not participate in anything if it is having a negative effect on your GPA. Lastly, do not forget to ascertain the necessary information from the experience and record it in your log. Everyone's experiences section will be different and that is completely okay. This is an opportunity to differentiate yourself and show who you truly are. If you follow your passions and interests, success will follow.

Chapter 5

The MCAT

So, what exactly is the Medical College Admissions Test or, as it is better known, the MCAT? Aside from knowing that they need a good score on the MCAT, many pre-med students are relatively unfamiliar with the test. If this is you, do not worry as we will cover how the MCAT is structured, how well medical schools expect you to perform on the MCAT, and some tips on how to prepare for the test itself in this chapter. However, this book is geared towards gaining acceptance into medical school not acing the MCAT, so while we will be discussing the MCAT, it is only in general terms. As you begin to prepare for the MCAT, you will need to go into much greater detail than described here.

A good MCAT score and GPA are the most important parts of your application, so this chapter is extremely important. While it is possible to get into medical school with a subpar MCAT score, having a great MCAT score will almost guarantee you interest from medical schools. Aside from gaining the interest of medical schools, a good MCAT score can also be used to compensate for a GPA that is less than desired. Doing well on the MCAT can show medical schools that you are able to comprehend and apply any topic that you may have earned a lower grade in. However, do not become overwhelmed by the pressure to do well on the MCAT. If you employ the strategies that we are going to discuss in this chapter and use proper planning, you will succeed on the MCAT.

While the exact structure and content of the test can be complicated and complex, it is not necessary to know many of the intricacies until you begin preparing for the exam. We will only go over the basics that you need to know while planning your journey. You will likely have more time to learn the nitty gritty details of the MCAT when you are closer to taking the test. In general, the test is composed of 4 sections: chemical and physical foundations of biological science (59 questions, 95 mins), critical analysis and reasoning skills (53 questions, 90 mins), biological and biochemical foundations of living systems (59 questions, 95 mins), and psychological, social, and biological foundations of behavior (59 questions, 95 mins). This is the order that you will be tested. You will be given an optional 10-minute break after each section and a 30-minute break for lunch after the CARS section. Each of these sections are scored independently and their sum is used to give you an overall score. The score for each section is between 118 and 132, so as you can deduce, your overall score on the MCAT will fall between 472 and 528. The test is scored on a bell curve with a mean score of 500. The sections are quite broad and consist of various topics. A list of each section and the topics covered is given here:

Chemical and Physical Foundations:

-General Chemistry

-Biochemistry

-Physics

-Organic Chemistry

-Biology

Critical Analysis and Reasoning Skills (CARS):

-Does not test any specific area of science in particular. Instead, it is aimed at determining your levels of comprehension and reasoning

Biological and Biochemical Foundations:

-Biology

-Biochemistry

-General Chemistry

-Organic Chemistry

Psychological, Social, and Biological Foundations of Behavior:

-Psychology

-Sociology

-Biology

In general, the MCAT will test your knowledge through the reading of passages and answering multiple choice questions. Each section of the MCAT will have multiple passages and each passage will be followed by passage-based questions. The exact number of passage-based questions related to each individual passage will vary. Generally, the passages that are followed by fewer questions are easier than those followed by many questions. In addition to passage-based questions, every section, except for CARS, will contain some standalone questions that test topics different from those of the passages. These standalone questions will draw on your previous knowledge of the subjects and the answer has nothing to do with any of the material in the passages.

That sums up the basics of the MCAT and, as stated before, this is not a guide to acing the MCAT. The general overview provided consists of everything that you need to know before preparing for the test. Once your test day gets closer and you begin to prepare, you will need to gain more of an understanding of the test. However, knowing the basics of the MCAT are necessary to understand the rest of the chapter.

Now that you have a basic understanding of the MCAT, we can discuss how good of a score is needed for acceptance into medical school. Similar to your GPA, the higher your MCAT score, the better, but a perfect score is by no means needed. Overall, you should shoot to be in the 75th percentile which translates to a 507 overall and or an average of almost 127 in each section. Although it is okay to not have equal scores across all sections of the test, you need to be leery of scoring too low in any individual section. While most medical schools only have a minimum requirement for the overall score, there are medical schools that have requirements for each individual section. You should aim to achieve no lower than a 125 in any individual section.

If you have taken the MCAT and did not earn a 507 or one of your sections was below a 125, this does not mean that you cannot become a physician. You have a few options depending on exactly what your score and GPA are. If your score is a 503 or better, I would advise you to continue to apply, especially if you have a good GPA and numerous great experiences. With a score in this range, I would advise that you retake the exam only if there is time, but do not postpone your application until next year because of a score in this range. If you scored between a 499 and a 502, I would advise that you retake the MCAT unless you have a great GPA and numerous high-quality experiences. While scores in this range are not horrible, they are not going to guarantee an interview. If you do not have time to retake the MCAT and need to apply in the current cycle, then by all means go for it. Do note, however, that in this score range, the other aspects of your application are going to be extremely important and you will need to do all of the little things amazingly well to earn a spot. Aside from perfecting the other areas of your application, I would advise you to cast a large net and apply to as many schools as possible. Lastly, if your score is below a 499, then you will probably need to retake the MCAT if you hope to go directly from undergrad to an American medical school. With a score below 499, it is very unlikely that you will be accepted to any medical school in the U.S. If you do not have time to retake the MCAT then you may want to consider applying to a Caribbean medical school or post-baccalaureate programs. We will go into more details on these options in 'Ch. 11, I Didn't get in... Now What?'

So, when should you take the MCAT and how long should you prepare for the exam? This is going to vary by when you want to apply to medical school and if you plan to take a gap year or not. If you plan to begin medical school immediately after graduation, then it is best to take the MCAT in the early to mid-summer before your senior year. However, if you plan to take a gap year then it is best to take the MCAT during the summer after you graduate. With both of these plans, you will begin applying to medical school immediately after you have taken the test. Taking the MCAT at one of these times will allow you some time to lightly prepare during the semester and then a short period of intense studying in the beginning of the summer before you take the test. Some applicants want to get a jump on other students and will take the test during the spring semester. While taking the test during the spring semester will allow plenty of time, if you need to retake the exam it will be next to impossible to properly prepare while enrolled full-time in classes. Preparing for the MCAT is a full-time job and should be treated as such. Anyone who takes the exam during the spring semester while enrolled in classes will most likely receive a lower score than if they had waited until the summer to take the test.

In general, you should attempt to spend 300 hours preparing for the MCAT. This is the national average for the amount of time that accepted students spend preparing for the MCAT.

While this may seem like a lot, if you consider that taking a single full-length practice test takes approximately 9 hours, you can see how you can arrive at 300 hours before you know it. Nonetheless, 300 hours is still quite a bit of time and this is why I suggest that you begin prepping for the test at least 2 months out. Before we discuss exactly what you should be doing during those 2 months prior, I want to point out that the MCAT, in theory, only tests material that you already know and is, therefore, a review.

Keeping this in mind, the most successful way of earning a great MCAT score is to prepare the entire time. Continually reviewing your past courses during your undergrad will help to keep the information fresh in your mind. This will benefit you greatly as the test nears and you don't have to waste time relearning material. This is why it is important to know what material is tested on the MCAT so that you know what courses to continually review. A popular way to continually review a class is to create a set of flashcards (up to 100) or a condensed set of notes (up to 5 pages) for each course that will be tested on the MCAT. There is likely to be 2 to 3 years between you completing some courses and taking the MCAT. If you do not revisit any of the concepts that you learned from the course during this time, you are likely to forget a great deal of what you learned.

One way to create flashcards or a condensed set of notes is to go through your notes for the entire course and work at identifying the key topics covered during the class and trans-lating them into your study tool. Try to avoid including too many small details as this is not the point of your study tool. Their purpose is to help you review the big ideas and key con-cepts of the course, not the nitty gritty details. You will have plenty of time to review the details when you begin intense preparation closer to the test. Overall, you want your study tool to be succinct yet comprehensive. Over time, you will create more and more of these tools and if they are too long in length, it will be hard to find the time to properly review them all. While condensing your notes or creating flashcards are probably the most popular, there are other options such as creating quizzes, diagrams, tables, outlines, videos, etc. The exact form of your review tool is not very important as long as it can carry out its desired function.

Once you have created these tools, it is important that you actually use them to review on a regular basis. After all, keeping the information current is the whole purpose. You should create a review schedule that is going to work best for your own individual needs. You are going to be busy during the year but should be able to find between 0.5-2 hours a week to dedicate to review. In the beginning, you may only have a single course or two to review and need to spend 30 mins a week. However, as you complete more courses, you will have more content to review. Thus, you will need to spend more time, closer to 2 hours per week reviewing. There are multiple ways to spread out your review time and it is best to try out a few different methods and see what works best for you. Some students may prefer to review multiple topics at once and complete all of their review in a single day. Others might prefer to spend 20 mins every other day focusing on a particular course. There are numerous ways to set up your review schedule. The important thing is that you find what works best for you and stick to it. This strategy will do you no good if you fail to create the study tools or execute your review schedule. Remember, this should be review and if you are spending large amounts of time relearning material, then you are not reviewing frequently enough.

While continual review is great for main ideas and key concepts, you will need to learn a great number of details for every subject. Aside from mastering the details, gaining some knowledge and skills with MCAT test-taking strategies will serve you well. This is what the 2 to 3 months before the MCAT should be used for. This time should be used for intense studying and preparation. The most effective way to prepare is to take an MCAT prep course, however, these can be extremely expensive and sometimes fill up quickly. If this is not an option then I would advise that you buy a set of books that complement an MCAT course and work through them by yourself. These courses and prep books will go into much greater detail on the MCAT and how to obtain a great score. As the test nears, make sure that you take numerous full-length practice tests and attempt to mimic the real testing experience as much as possible. The test is mentally taxing and you do not want the first time you take a test of that length and difficulty to be on test day.

This is by no means comprehensive coverage of how to prepare for the MCAT but simply a guide as to what you should be doing in the years leading up to the test. This general overview should serve you well in gaining an understanding of the test and its contents. Being familiar with the test is the first step in preparing successfully. Beyond simply knowing what the test contains, you should now have some knowledge on how well you need to perform and the options that scores in certain ranges will provide you. The MCAT is extremely important, but as with most aspects of getting into medical school, it can be conquered through proper preparation and execution of your plan. Creating study tools that allow for continuous review throughout your undergraduate years is a great start. Continually reviewing material will allow you to fully utilize the period of intense preparation before your exam. This intense time can now be dedicated to learning the details and improving MCAT test-taking strategies and skills.

Chapter 6

Personal Statement

The personal statement is your chance to tell your story. It is an opportunity to tell not only what you have done, but how it has shaped you as a person and future physician. Essentially, you will detail the emotional side of your experiences and explain how they will make you a better physician in the future. A large majority of your application is simply checking boxes and listing activities without much room to touch on the emotional or personal side of things. This is your chance to show medical schools who you are and how you differ from the other applicants. The key is to demonstrate introspection and tell a story that goes beyond the experiences themselves. Whether you are detailing a specific activity or discussing your entire undergraduate career, this is your chance to expand on what you have done.

Before going any further, it is time to discuss how this section of the application is structured. Both the AMCAS and AACOMAS will have a large text box for you to write your personal statement. While it is possible to work on your personal statement in this text box, I would not advise it. It should take a considerable amount of time to construct your personal statement and you will need to have it edited and proofread at least once before submission. It is best to already have your personal statement completed by the time you are going to apply and then simply copy and paste your personal statement into the text box when it is time. The only major difference between the MD and DO application is the maximum number of characters allowed. The AMCAS has a limit of 5300 characters, while the AACOMAS has a limit of only 4500 characters. While this is not too large of a difference, it is important to note before beginning your statement. It is possible that your personal statement ends up meeting the requirements for both applications. However, it is more likely that you will need to produce a condensed form of your AMCAS statement for the AACOMAS. While some people may tell you that it is necessary to write different statements for each type of application, this may not be true. Unless you explicitly state some sort of information that pertains to only MDs or DOs, this is not necessary.

The personal statement section of the application is not only unique in its content but also in its level of importance. The effect that a personal statement has on your application can be somewhat trivial. The best personal statement in the world will not guarantee you acceptance, but a poorly written personal statement will most certainly remove you from consideration. Writing your personal statement is often a balancing act between creating good enough work that you are not automatically rejected but not spending too much time on your statement that other areas of your application suffer. While many students place an extremely high priority on their personal statement, this section of the application is often overrated. While you do not need to compose a masterpiece of a personal statement, it must still be good enough to draw interest and not receive an automatic rejection. However, if your GPA or MCAT score is not where they need to be, then you will need to put more effort into your personal statement.

With academics lacking, a great personal statement is a must to compensate for the weaknesses in your application.

There are many different ways to structure and organize your personal statement. Some students will focus on a particular moment or experience, while others will give more of a broad overview of their entire undergrad experience. Exactly what you discuss and how you structure your personal statement is completely up to you. However, in order to write a great personal statement, you will need to answer these 4 questions:

1. Why do you want to become a physician?

2. What have you done during your undergrad to explore and expand your interest?

3. How have these experiences changed or shaped you?

4. Explain how your experiences and their effects on you personally will make you a great physician in the future?

These are simply prompts for writing your personal statement and should not serve as your outline. Do not simply answer these questions in a report style that is similar to something you would produce for your English class. Your personal statement is a free-flowing expression of yourself and your individual experiences. While this may seem abstract and not provide much detail, that is the whole point. There is no outline or template for a perfect personal statement. As the name states, it needs to be personal. It needs to be unique. If you are having trouble answering these questions, I have listed some alternative questions that you can address. Answering these questions should help you to form a more developed and well-rounded answer to the previous questions.

1b. What is your motivation? What was your deciding moment in choosing to become a physician? What is your inspiration for wanting to become a physician?

2b. What is the most memorable moment of your undergrad? What was your favorite experience? How did you spend most of your time?

3b. What was your most life-changing experience? How are you different from when you began college? What is the most important life-lesson you learned?

4b. What will make you a good physician? What do you have in common with a good physician?

The uniqueness of your personal statement is vital to its success. You want to use unique statements whenever possible. Try to avoid using statements that could hold true for any applicant. Instead, use statements that only pertain to you. A simple and effective way to do this is through providing detailed examples that only pertain to you.

"I am a hardworking and intelligent individual who is passionate about helping others".

This statement can pertain to anyone. There is nothing unique about this sentence, nothing that makes it personal. This statement could be written by any applicant. However, if we expand this sentence to:

"I am a hardworking and intelligent individual who is passionate about helping others. This past summer, I took an EMT course and now work as an EMT on nights and weekends. I truly enjoy working as an EMT as it allows me to administer care to individuals in need."

By expanding on the original statement, we are able to make it more unique and personal. The statement now only pertains to us, it can no longer refer to every applicant. We have demonstrated your intelligence by mentioning the extra course you took during the summer. We have demonstrated your work ethic through mentioning that you work as an EMT in addition to school. Lastly, we show your passion for helping others by mentioning the enjoyment that you get in providing care.

As with most topics in this book, the key is to get an early start and not procrastinate. You should begin working on your personal statement the semester before the summer you plan to apply. By starting your personal statement early, you will have plenty of time to outline and construct a great personal statement without being rushed. If you wait until the summer to begin working on your personal statement, you will certainly be pressured. This pressure will arise due to the time constraints. There is immense pressure to submit your application as early as possible, as this will increase your chances. There is also a limited amount of time available to work on your personal statement. Most of your time this summer should be spent preparing for the MCAT and filling out the rest of the application.

Aside from relieving pressures, working on your statement during the semester allows you to access all of the resources that your school has available. The key resource here is your pre-med advisor. While you can still communicate with your pre-med advisor during the summer, it is much easier and more efficient to meet face to face. Also, your pre-med advisor is going to be extremely busy during the summer, as this is when students will be applying to medical school. Your pre-med advisor should be able to help you generate ideas, outline your statement, and proofread or edit for errors in content or format. Most likely, they will have read hundreds of personal statements and should have a wealth of knowledge to help you construct a great personal statement. Another resource available to you is the university's English department. Whether you receive help from a previous English professor or a student who volunteers in the writing or resource center, it is important to have your statement edited for errors in grammar, syntax, etc. Again, this is much easier and more efficient if you are physically on campus. The last and final resource that you have is your fellow pre-med students, past and present. Don't be afraid to talk to your peers about their personal statements or ask to see a copy of a friend's who is now a medical student. Most medical students remember being in your shoes and are more than willing to help. We are all in this together and it is important to help one another. Remember to pay it forward when you are in medical school or a physician and help those trying to follow in your footsteps. While it can be helpful to discuss or read personal statements of your peers, it is important to create your own. Old personal statements can offer some help but make sure to limit their influence. You are an individual who is completely different from everyone else. Copying someone else's thoughts, ideas, and style are not likely to work as well for you.

While it may seem like starting to write your statements 6 months prior to applying is a bit extreme, I promise you that it isn't. Working on your statement throughout the semester and having it done by summer will save you huge amounts of time and stress. The summer that you are taking the MCAT and applying is already going to be challenging enough. It will be a huge weight off your shoulders if you have your personal statement finished and simply need to copy and paste it into the text box.

Make the most of your personal statement but do not put forth an unnecessarily excessive amount of effort. Hopefully, you are not too stressed with the idea of writing a personal statement. Most people find composing their personal statement one of the most enjoyable parts of the application as it allows you a chance for introspection and to tell your story. This is your chance to demonstrate all that you have gained in the past few years. So, enjoy it and make the most of this opportunity.

Chapter 7

Recommendation Letters

The last piece of the primary application are the letters of recommendation. This can often be the most stressful part of the primary application as it is the portion that students have the least control over. While it can be difficult to put all of your faith in someone else, especially in such an important matter, there is no need to worry. There are certain steps that you can take in the months leading up to the application that will guarantee a good outcome. This chapter will look at the importance of recommendation letters, how to obtain them, and who to ask.

Of all the sections on the primary application, the recommendation letters are the least important. Nonetheless, you still need them in your application, though they generally hold little importance. Similar to the personal statement, a great letter of recommendation by itself will not get you an acceptance. However, if your letter of recommendation is actually a letter of disapproval, then you will most likely be rejected. While the exact words the author uses in the letter are not very important, it is important that those words are positive. The low amount of importance placed on letters of recommendation is in large part due to the standardization of these letters. Almost every letter will list good qualities or attributes that the student possesses and describe what they have accomplished. In general, every letter describes how great you are. While it is important to have someone willing to say such nice things about you, there is hardly any meaningful difference between recommendation letters. The positive letters have very little difference but if the author begins detailing how awful of a person you are, the admissions committee will take notice. If someone writes you a negative letter of recommendation, then you will most likely be rejected. Believe it or not, some authors will accept the offer to write a recommendation letter and then project the student in a negative light. This is why it is imperative that you know the author well and are sure of how they feel about you. Regardless of what your recommendation letter contains or who writes it, the letter needs to represent you in a positive light.

When you arrive at this section of the application, there will be some relief as this section of the primary application is the easiest to fill out. Here, you will enter each author's individual information, at which point, the process leaves your hands as the application service sends the author an email. This email will contain all of the specific information and instructions needed to complete the application. It is best to ask the authors of your letters to send you a confirmation email stating that they have received an email from the application service. The last thing you want is for the email to be filtered to the author's junk folder where it will eventually be lost or deleted. In addition to confirming that the author received the email from the application service, you should stress to the author the importance of following the instructions exactly. This is imperative as any deviations from the instructions can result in the letter being delayed or not accepted. While the processes for the AMCAS and AACOMAS work the same, you will need separate letters for each type of application. It is okay to use the same letters on both types of applications. However, make sure that the author is aware that they will have to submit the letter twice, once to AMCAS and once to AACOMAS.

After the authors have submitted their letters of recommendation, the application service will review and approve the letters. Now the control shifts back to the applicant as you are able to select specific letters and assign them to specific schools. However, you will not be allowed to view the letters, you will only receive a confirmation that they have been received.

Knowing exactly what letters to assign to what schools can sometimes be difficult. The requirements concerning letters of recommendation will vary from medical school to medical school. It is best to look at each individual school's website or contact their office of admissions to determine exactly what is needed. In general, you want to submit between 3-5 letters from a diverse group of authors. Even though you may have more than 5 letters of recommendation, I would not advise that you send any more. As discussed earlier, letters of recommendation hold very little weight and by increasing the number of letters submitted beyond 5, you are more likely to hurt yourself than help. It is highly unlikely that the 6th letter or 7th letter will contain some new piece of information that was not already discussed in the first 5 letters. Thus, there is not much of an incentive to send excessive letters as the additional letters could contain information that would hurt your chances. Overall, when it comes to assigning letters to specific schools, it is best to follow their requirements and possibly add 1 or 2 additional letters but no more.

Due to the variation in the requirements of recommendation letters, it is best to have a diverse pool of authors. Simply having 3 science professors write you letters of recommendation will not suffice. You should attempt to gather a letter of recommendation from at least 1 physician (MD or DO), 2 science professors, 1 non-science professor, and 1 employer/manager. This should serve as the bare minimum and it is highly encouraged that you gather 2 to 3 more letters. Any advisor, a supervisor of an organization, or any other superior are great choices for these additional letters. The additional letters can also come from any of the groups previously listed. Regardless of who you choose to write your letters of recommendation, make sure that you have a professional relationship with them. Most medical schools are not interested or intrigued by personal references, i.e. family members or family friends

While having stellar letters of recommendation is not absolutely necessary, it will certainly not hurt your chances. With that said, the key to obtaining a great letter of recommendation is to know the author very well. The better the relationship that you and the author have, the better the odds are of you receiving a great letter of recommendation. This can sometimes be hard to achieve as it takes time to develop a lasting relationship and as you have probably already noticed, time can be in short supply while preparing for the application process. Perhaps you developed a great relationship with your general chemistry professor during your freshman year but haven't taken one of their courses since. As you can imagine, it can be quite challenging for this professor to write you a good letter of recommendation years later due to the time that has passed since you last interacted. However, you can overcome this by staying in constant contact with this professor. Staying in touch is the key to developing a good relationship and receiving a good letter of recommendation. There are many ways to stay in touch such as writing to your professors at the end of every semester to fill them in or stopping by their office hours every once in a while to catch up. Some people even write previous professors birthday or holiday emails. Whatever method you choose, it is important to keep in touch and keep your professor up to date. Also, this does not only apply to professors, it is a good idea to keep in touch with anyone who you might ask to write a letter of recommendation, i.e. physicians, managers, advisors, etc.

Once the time has come to officially ask someone to write you a letter of recommendation, there are a couple of questions that you want to ask them. First, "Would you be willing to write a letter of recommendation for me?". Assessing if someone is willing to write a letter for you is the first step. The last thing you want is to have someone writing you a letter that they were unenthusiastic about. Even though that may turn out okay, the letter will not be of the same quality as someone who is ready and willing. The second question you should ask is, "Do you feel that you are in a position to write a good letter of recommendation for me?". This question is aimed at determining how well the person knows you and what they think of you. If someone does not know you well enough to compose a good letter or if they think poorly of you, this question will give them a way out. Similar to the first question, we do not want someone writing us a letter of recommendation if it will not be of an acceptable caliber.

Assuming that they answered yes to the first 2 questions, it is important that you take this next step. You should come to an agreement on an exact date by which they will have the recommendation completed. Many of the authors of these letters are extremely busy individuals and writing a letter of recommendation can often get pushed back. By getting them to agree to a deadline, you have now gained the ability to contact them if the application service has not notified you of the letter's arrival by the deadline. Without this agreement, you may find yourself with the dilemma of wanting an update regarding your recommendation but not wanting to be a nuisance to the author. While it is completely fine to send a reminder to the author after the deadline has passed, it is important to remain polite, respectful, and professional. This will guarantee that the author still writes you a positive letter.

In addition to these questions, it is generally a good idea to have some form of a resume or CV prepared for the authors. Even though you may have a close relationship with a potential author, they are often not aware of everything that you are doing. Providing them with a resume or CV will help to make them aware of any experiences that you have gained outside of their own personal involvement with you. Hopefully, your author will not need a resume to write you a letter of recommendation but it never hurts. You should be updating your resume or CV on a regular basis anyway so there should not be much effort needed here. Providing your recommender with this extra information will only help to improve their letter of recommendation.

Even though letters of recommendation are one of the least important sections of your application, they are still, nevertheless, important. While it is not necessary that you receive an amazing letter written by the surgeon general of the United States, it is important that there is a diverse group of people willing to vouch for you. Simply creating this group of supporters during your undergrad is simply not enough and you must also stay in contact, keeping them up to date. Building the type of relationship necessary for an author to write you a good letter of recommendation takes time and effort. Putting in this time and effort before it is time to apply will once again save you time and stress. Getting a good start on developing these relationships, working to maintain them, and providing the author with a resume or CV will guarantee that you receive outstanding letters of recommendation.

Part II:

Time to APPLY

You are now familiar with the application and all of its components, as well as the steps that you should be taking in the years leading up to applying (For a free example of a timeline, visit MasteringMedicalEducation. wordpress.com). At this point, you should have taken all of the steps necessary before you apply but this is only the beginning. Now it is the time to fill out the primary application, complete secondary applications, and attend interviews. Completing the primary application at this point should be relatively simple as you are, more or less, filling in the boxes on the application. The next portions of the application process are less well-known as many people focus on the elements of the primary application but that is only half of the process. Part II will discuss everything that goes on after you have finished filling in the boxes on your application.

Chapter 8

Choosing a Medical School

W hen I began applying to medical school, I was so focused on simply getting in that when it came time to decide which schools to apply to, I had a hard time. I discovered that I knew very little about the differences between medical schools. Due to my lack of familiarity with medical schools, I had absolutely no idea what I was looking for. Most people put forth so much effort into just getting in that they do not take the time to find a good fit. Here are a few things that I wish I had known to consider when I was applying to medical schools.

When it comes to applying to medical school, the first decision that you must make is on the type of medical school that you want to attend. In general, there are 3 options: Doctor of Medicine (MD), Doctor of Osteopathy (DO), or a Caribbean medical school. You may choose to apply to only 1 type or all 3. Applying to more than 1 type is encouraged as it will not hurt your chances, but do not apply to any school that you ultimately would never attend as it is simply a waste of time and resources. All 3 types of medical schools are great options and there are numerous exceptional physicians who have developed their skills and knowledge from each of the 3 types. Attending 1 type of school truly has no bearing on how successful you will be in the future, that is all up to you and the effort that you put forth. In almost any clinic, hospital, or other healthcare setting, you will most likely see a mix of physicians, from all 3 types of schools, performing the same tasks. Becoming an exceptional physician is determined by the extent to which you benefit others, not what letters appear after your name. While the destination upon graduation from any of these types of medical schools will be the same, there are some very small differences.

Osteopathic medicine is a relatively new field of medicine that has expanded rapidly in the past 40 years. DO schools follow the same curriculum as the MD schools, but also learn more holistic techniques such as manual manipulations. These manipulations are one of the hallmarks of holistic care. DO physicians tend to look at the entire body (holistic) instead of the individual organ or region affected when treating a patient. Although DOs tend to take a more holistic approach, that does not exclude them from being able to specialize in any area of medicine.

In general, Caribbean medical schools accept lower GPAs and MCAT scores than schools in the states. If you are unsure of whether or not you will be accepted into medical school, I would advise that you apply to a couple of Caribbean medical schools as a backup plan. This way, if you do not get into any medical schools in the U.S., you do not have to take a year off to improve your application and can thus begin school as planned. Even though these schools are in a different country, they are affiliated with U.S. medical institutions and you will be allowed to practice in the U.S. upon completion. They are often a great alternative for those who do not get accepted into their school of choice. However, these schools do not use the AMCAS or AACOMAS application service. Thus, if you are interested in applying it is best to visit the individual school's website and go from there. But only apply if you are serious about attending.

Caribbean medical schools have some subtle differences between them but, overall, they follow the same path. You will spend your first year and a half to 2 years in the Caribbean at whichever institution you choose to attend. This time will largely be spent in the classroom learning the material needed for the board exams. After you have finished the material, you will most likely take a board exam and upon achieving a successful score, you will begin clinical rotations in the U.S. at a number of sites throughout the country. Alternatively, some schools may have you rotate through a few clinical rotations in the U.S. before taking your board exam. Regardless of what route your school takes after you have spent your time in the Caribbean learning the material, you will finish your education stateside. Upon completion of the program, your graduation may be back in the Caribbean or in the U.S. This will vary from school to school.

As a student at a Caribbean medical school, you are still eligible to apply for all of the same residencies that medical students in the states are eligible for. While there is ABSO-LUTELY nothing wrong with attending a Caribbean medical school, it is no secret that they have less stringent requirements for acceptance. Due to this, it is important that you put forth your best effort on the board exams in order to help level your playing field. With that being said, your success as a physician will be determined by your own effort, not by where you attended medical school.

Aside from the type of medical school that you would like to attend, another important consideration is the different number and types of programs offered by the medical school. Some schools offer fast track (3-year programs) for those wishing to enter primary care. Some pre-med students know that they want to practice primary care and have no interest in specializing. There is nothing wrong with this, especially as there is currently a shortage of primary care physicians and the deficit is only going to increase in the coming years. The last 2 years of medical schools (years 3 & 4) consist of clinical rotations through various specialties and away electives in specialties of your choice. The goal of these years is to not only gain knowledge but exposure to numerous different areas of medicine to assist in choosing a specialty. However, for those who already know that they wish to practice primary care, some of these rotations and electives can be seen as unnecessary. This is why some medical schools now offer a fast track for those wishing to pursue primary care. These programs generally take 3 years to complete. While these programs vary, in general, some of the more specialized portions of years 3 & 4 are eliminated as they do not pertain to primary care. This allows students to shave a year off of their journey to becoming a practicing physician. These programs are becoming more popular in recent years and are a great option for those who have a passion for primary care.

Other schools offer dual degree programs such as MD-PhD, MD-MPH, and MD-MBA. While these are usually secondary considerations, if you are interested in a career beyond practicing, these are great opportunities. A dual degree is a great option for students looking to become involved beyond simply practicing. For those students who are very interested in research, an MD-PhD is a great option. These programs are for students who, in general, wish to become medical researchers. As a medical researcher, you would spend most of your time working on projects and very little, if any, time practicing. An MD-MPH is a great option for students who have an interest in public health. This is a way for students to gain knowledge in public health and is often a great option for those physicians who look to become more involved in community initiatives such as awareness programs, educational programs, community support groups, etc. While many MD-MPH physicians spend a significant amount of time working on initiatives, they still practice frequently. The MD-MBA degree is geared towards students who have an interest in how medicine and business interact. The MD-MBA degree can lead to a plethora of careers; owning a private practice, hospital administration, Dean of a medical school, and CEO of a biotechnology company are just a few of the many options available to those with both degrees.

The final consideration for choosing a medical school is perhaps the least important but still needs to be mentioned. If you plan to pursue a career in research or research is very important to you, then it is important to consider the medical school's research reputation. It is important that if you have a passion for research that the school meets or exceeds your own passion. Without the equality of passions, it is highly unlikely that your expectations and goals in terms of research will be met. Likewise, if research is not of the upmost importance to you then there is nothing to worry about. All schools will provide their students with some sort of opportunity for research.

While interacting with medical schools via the application process, interview day, or second look day, make sure to take note of the culture and atmosphere of the school. These are some of the intangibles that can play a major role in finding a good fit for yourself. There are definite differences in culture between medical schools. Make sure to choose a school that feels like a good fit. Sometimes the school that is the best fit for you might not be the most prestigious, closest to home, or the one that you have always dreamed of. Make sure to always have an open mind when visiting a school. With this being said, finding a good fit is imperative to your success. Some schools breed a culture of immense competition while others are more team-based. Immense competition can bring out the best in some students but could also debilitate another, yet fully capable, student. Finding an environment that best suits you will do more for you in the long-term than choosing to attend a school simply for its reputation or national rank.

Although gaining an acceptance should be your number one priority, it is important to find the right medical school for you. Hopefully, these topics will help to guide you once the time comes to select a medical school.

Chapter 9

Secondary Applications

After you have completed the primary application and selected which medical schools to apply to, you should begin receiving secondary applications. Most of the secondary applications will require you to submit between 1 to 5 essays and possibly some other information that is not contained in the primary application. Even though these essays are relatively short, under 500 words, they will vary from school to school and you could easily end up having to write 20 unique short essays. With this being said, it important that you do not procrastinate as it is very easy to fall behind and end up submitting subpar secondary essays.

While receiving a secondary can mean that the medical school has some level of interest in you, it is not the best indicator. Exactly who receives a secondary application will vary among medical schools, many medical schools simply send every applicant a secondary or at least every applicant who meets their minimum GPA and MCAT requirements. Secondary applications are the first chance that the medical school has to gather the information that they want. Up until this point in time, medical schools only have access to the same information as every other medical school. Medical schools can now obtain additional and unique information from you regarding whatever subject or area they are interested in. When applying, you can expect to pay an average of $75-$100 per secondary application. While some applicants can apply for a fee waiver, these secondary application fees can become quite expensive for others.

The essay prompts or topics are going to vary from school to school but there are still some ways to prepare. While not guaranteed, some essay prompts are somewhat standard. A potential secondary essay prompt will ask what interests you in their school in particular. For these essays, it is a good idea to research the school and attempt to identify unique aspects of the school that you can relate to and are able to articulate. Another potential prompt will ask something such as, "What will make you a good physician in the future or why do you want to become a physician?". While these are most likely topics that you covered in your personal statement, make sure to respond to this question in a new way. It will do you no good to answer the question in the same way twice.

Secondary applications are one of the easier parts of the application process but they can be costly and time-consuming, requiring you to plan accordingly. The uniqueness of essay prompts and time needed to research the medical school can end up taking a considerable amount of time, so it is best to not procrastinate. Complete your secondary applications in a timely manner and then prepare for the waiting game. After you have submitted your secondary applications, you could end up waiting anywhere from 1 week to 4 months before hearing back from a school regarding an interview or a rejection.

Chapter 10

Interview Day

fter your secondary applications are received, medical schools will begin to evaluate your entire application and, at this point, they will either offer you an interview or send you a rejection. In this chapter, we will discuss what a typical interview day will look like as well as how to properly prepare. Beyond what to expect, we will also discuss what being invited for an interview means and the next steps in the application process. The knowledge gained in this chapter will help to alleviate the unknown and prepare you to be successful on interview day.

The first step is to schedule the interview. Medical schools will offer numerous interview days throughout the interview season allowing you to choose the best date for you. Make sure to select a day where you are able to miss classes and not a day where you are supposed to take an exam. It is important to finish strong and pass all your classes during your final year, as medical schools will require you to send in a final transcript consisting of all classes taken before you may begin. While you do not have to pick the first available date, it is advantageous to interview earlier in the process. Most schools admit students on a rolling basis so the earlier you interview, the more spots available. As the year progresses and fewer and fewer spots are available, medical schools become more selective.

Once you have selected a date, it is best to begin making travel accommodations as soon as possible. Accommodations will vary largely between medical schools due to factors such as travel time, distance, interview check-in time, etc. Interview day is likely to be somewhat stressful and having many of the details figured out ahead of time is a great way to alleviate some of this stress and anxiety.

Another area that causes some applicants stress is the topic of what to wear. First impressions are an incredibly powerful tool when it comes to an interview. While great attire will by no means get you an acceptance, wearing an outfit that is too revealing or not professional could go a long way in hurting your chances. Exactly what you wear does not matter as long as it is professional and well-kept. Many men often choose to wear the standard black suit but if you would prefer to wear a blue or gray suit then by all means go for it. The same is true for women, do not feel as though you must wear a black dress or a suit. Feel free to express yourself and wear whatever you like as long as it is professional. Choosing something different from the norm can make you stand out to interviewers but make sure that you do not stray too far from the norm as this may turn them off.

The last preparation that you can make before the interview is to practice sample questions and review your application, primary and secondary. While it is impossible to know exactly what questions the school will ask you, spending time answering practice questions is a great way to prepare yourself. Many interviewers will have access to your application and will often formulate questions that stem from your application. It is important that you are familiar with your application so that your answers line up with the information in your application. For a free list of practice questions, visit Master-ingMedicalEducation.wordpress.com.

While the exact schedule and format of interview day will vary among medical schools, there are some standard activities. Typically, the interview day will begin in the morning and finish in the evening. There are numerous other activities that you will partake in aside from the interview itself. The exact order, duration, and topics covered during the day will vary between medical schools. Every medical school will schedule a few hours for the interviewees to gather information on the school. You will usually gather this information through listening to presentations. These presentations generally cover topics such as financial aid, curriculum, school calendar, extra-curricular opportunities, etc. Another portion of the day will typically be spent taking a tour of the campus and interacting with current students. Feel free to ask the current students any questions that you have as they are usually your best bet at receiving a candid answer. The final portion of the day will be spent interviewing.

The exact format, duration, and number of interviews will vary from school to school but, in general, there are 2 formats. The first format is a traditional format where you will provide answers to questions asked of you by either a single person or panel. These are usually longer in length and ask more traditional questions. The second type of interview conducted by medical schools is the multiple mini interview (MMI). The MMI format is gaining popularity in recent years. In general, an MMI consists of numerous short interviews, usually under 10 minutes. The MMI will usually have many stations that interviewees rotate through. The topics covered or questions asked at each station will vary greatly from one another. The first station may ask why you want to become a physician, while the next station involves the interviewee partaking in a role-play or skit. While these are the most common interview formats, they allow for many different variations. It is best to contact each individual school before attending the interview to determine the exact format of their interview.

Once the interview day has concluded, it is once again time to play the waiting game. The exact amount of time between your interview and a decision will vary for each school and depend on the time of year. Things such as winter break can sometimes delay decision announcements. After your interview has concluded, the interviewer(s) will fill out a form evaluating your answers and overall performance. This form will then be added to your application file. Your application is now complete and will move on to the final phase. The completed application will then make its way to the admissions committee. These committees normally consist of faculty members, administration, physicians, and other community members who are involved in the medical school. The committee will collectively evaluate each individual application and arrive at a decision. In general, there are 3 decisions that the admissions committee can make: Acceptance, waitlist, or decline.

If you are granted an acceptance, congratulations! There is nothing wrong with accepting multiple acceptances and narrowing it down to a single school later on. However, some schools do require that you make a non-refundable deposit in order to hold your seat. This cost is simply something to be aware of as you move forward.

If you are told that you were placed on the waitlist, there is no need to immediately fret. A decent percentage of the final class will consist of students from the waitlist. Many people who are accepted immediately will occupy multiple acceptances across numerous schools. As time goes on, they will reduce the number of spots taken and free up space for others. While being on the waitlist is not anyone's first choice, it still allows for the chance of an acceptance.

The final outcome would be to receive a denial from the school. This is an unfortunate result and, hopefully, you have other interviews scheduled. While this is obviously not the outcome that you hoped for, it is important that you treat this as an opportunity to learn. Try to reflect back on the day of the interview and determine areas where you could improve. Making small changes could go a long way in your future interviews. You should also reflect on your strengths. It is equally as important to figure out what you are doing right and continue those actions and behaviors.

Interview day is the final step in applying to medical school and perhaps the most important. This will most likely be one of the most stressful days in the process but it is important to relax and remain calm. As with almost everything in this book, making proper preparations ahead of time can go a long way in relieving stress and increasing chances of success. Making proper accommodations, practicing potential questions, and determining the interview format should all help prepare you for what to expect. After the interview day is over, the waiting game continues and if you have followed the steps outlined in this book, then good news is most likely on the way. However, if for some reason good news did not make its way to you, there is still hope. The next chapter discusses some of your potential options if you did not get an acceptance.

Chapter 11

I didn't get in ... Now what?

If interview season has come and gone and you have not been granted an acceptance, do not fret. While this is obviously not the outcome that you wanted, it does not mean that you have no chance of becoming a physician. Medical schools are filled with students who had to apply multiple times in order to gain an acceptance. Just because you were not granted an acceptance does not mean that your dream is over. There are still many options for you to pursue.

The first thing to determine after not being granted an acceptance is whether or not you wish to reapply to medical school. While many will choose to reapply, there are others who, for whatever reason, will choose another path. You do not need to be a physician in order to help individuals through medicine. There are numerous other occupations in the healthcare field which can be just as satisfying as a physician.

If you have decided to reapply then the following will help make sure the final result turns out much better for you. The most important thing that you can do after not getting accepted is to NOT take the year off. It is extremely important that you are productive while reapplying, do NOT take the year off. If you do nothing to improve your application then you will end up with the same result. You should begin improving your chances of gaining an acceptance by identifying any weaknesses in your application and working to strengthen them.

Aside from evaluating your application on your own, most medical schools who invited you for an interview are willing to discuss your application with you. While discussing your entire application with you, the medical schools will identify any areas in which they would like to see improvement. While some of the suggestions may be school-specific, there should also be commonalities between medical schools. If you were not granted an opportunity to interview with a medical school, then it is best to meet with your pre-med advisor. They will most likely have no access to your application so you will need to print out a copy for them to review. Your pre-med advisor will also have no information regarding how you did in the interview, so it is important that you are honest with them so that they can provide meaningful advice. If you are not honest with your pre-med advisor or do not give them access to your application, they will not be able to help you to their fullest capabilities. Despite some of these limitations, your pre-med advisor should still be able to give you plenty of constructive advice on how to improve your application for the next cycle.

In general, there are 3 areas where most pre-medical students need to improve if they were not granted an acceptance; MCAT score, experience, and interview skills. While these may not apply to you, most students will have been rejected due to a weakness in at least 1 of these areas. The only thing worse than actually taking the MCAT is prepping for the MCAT and while nobody wants to do either again, the fact of the matter is, you will most likely need to improve your score if you want an acceptance. When preparing to take the MCAT for a second time, it is imperative that you take it even more seriously than you did the first time. If you prepare for the MCAT in the same way, you are likely to get the same result. At this point, you should be somewhat comfortable with the exam and strategies that you need to employ and should be able to focus most of your time on mastering the material. It is important to identify your weakest areas of the MCAT and spend the most time on them. While it feels good to review material that we are comfortable with and get practice questions right, this is often the most inefficient way to study. Even though it may not be the most immediately satisfying, spend most of your time on the difficult topics and it will pay off in the end.

A lack of experience is another common area of weakness within an application. As we discussed, there are 3 types of experience and while perhaps you are strong enough in 2 of the 3, there could still be much room for improvement in the final area. If you do not have any research experience, I would highly recommend that you spend some time over the course of the next year in a lab. Research experience is the most highly regarded, and a lack thereof could be a major factor holding you back. Regardless of the type of experience that you are lacking, it will behoove you to strengthen it when reapplying.

The last common area of weakness is the interview itself. If you have phenomenal primary and secondary applications yet you still did not receive an acceptance, this is most likely due to your interview. Being granted numerous interviews while not receiving any acceptances is usually an indicator of poor interview skills. While having poor interview skills is an issue, as mentioned before, most medicals schools who interviewed you are willing to meet with you regarding why they choose not to grant you an acceptance. This is a great opportunity to determine exactly what went wrong in the interview and determine how to rectify your mistakes before the next application cycle is over. Perhaps you were too nervous, unprepared for the questions, or failed to develop a good rapport with your interviewer. No matter what the case was it is important to spend time preparing to avoid making the same mistakes again.

Another option if you are not granted an acceptance into medical school but still wish to become a physician is to apply for a Master's or Post-Baccalaureate program through the medical school or its associated university. This is a great way to network within the medical school and prepare to attend. Many medical schools have programs for students who they are interested in yet they do not think are quite ready for the rigors of medical schools. These programs often last a year and give the student a chance to strengthen their basic science knowledge in preparation for medical school. Also, upon successful completion of many of these programs, students are granted an automatic acceptance into the medical school the following year. These programs do vary between medical schools and it is best to inquire about specifics such as program type (Master's or Post-Bacc), how to apply, cost, duration, and other factors at each school individually.

We've discussed your options if you have decided to reapply but this is not the decision that all denied applicants choose. Some applicants have applied later in life, others have already reapplied and yet to receive an acceptance, regardless of the reason why, not all applicants decide to apply again. If you decide to no longer apply to medical school, there other jobs in the healthcare field that you are well qualified for due to your attempt at medical school. These jobs are all great options for those who hope to have a positive effect through healthcare. Five great options for continuing your education and working in healthcare are nursing school, physician assistant (PA) school, optometry school, a Master's in public health (MPH), and a Master's in hospital administration (MHA).

The curriculum and experiences that you gathered on your path towards applying to medical school will transfer well into any of these fields. Some of these educational paths will allow you the opportunity to treat patients and others allow for you to make a change in a more hands-off way. While this list is by no means all-inclusive these are all popular options for those who are unable to earn an acceptance.

Attending nursing school is often a good option because of the breadth of work environments and opportunity for growth. As a nurse, you are able to care for patients in almost every healthcare setting. Although as a nurse you will not treat patients in the same manner as a physician, nurses have many opportunities to care for patients directly. Another benefit of becoming a nurse is the opportunity for growth. As a nurse, you have the opportunity to progress into careers such as a midwife, nurse anesthetist, or nurse practitioner (NP). While the downside of attending nursing school is the fact that upon graduation you will have earned another bachelor's degree and if you wish to progress to NP you could end up spending the same amount of time in school as if you were to become a physician. However, since you have an extremely strong science background some nursing schools will credit you with up to 2 years of nursing school. So, while becoming a nurse might not have been your original plan there are many parallels between nurses and physicians and it is a great career.

Becoming a PA is another great option for those who have decided to not reapply to medical school. As a PA, you are still able to treat patients and there are opportunities for specialization. Some PA's even perform surgeries. PA programs are generally 2 years long and, at the end, you will have earned a Master's degree. While a pre-med curriculum will prepare you very well to attend PA there are other requirements that you most likely will have to spend time in order to achieve. The first being that you will have to take the Graduate Records Examination (GRE). This exam is much shorter and, in general, easier than the MCAT. Some schools may accept an MCAT score in place of the GRE but most will require you to take it. In addition, most PA schools will require or recommend 500-1000 hours of healthcare experience. Hopefully, you already have some healthcare experience or perhaps you already have enough. Regardless of what the case is this is a large enough difference between medical applications that it should be noted. If it was extremely hard for you to accept that you will no longer become a physician then PA might be the best fit for you. Becoming a PA is probably the closest option to becoming a physician as you can treat patients on your own, perform surgery, and in most states, prescribe medicine.

Optometry school is yet another educational path that a pre-med curriculum will prepare you well for. As an optometrist, you will provide general care of the eyes and determine prescription strengths for glasses and contacts. Although optometrists are not able to provide the same level of care as an ophthalmologist, this is another great career that can enable you to care for patients. In order to become an optometrist, you will need to earn a Doctor of Optometry degree (O.D.). Earning this degree will take 4 years and you must earn a good score on the Optometry Admission Test (OAT) before you will be accepted.

Another great option for those who choose to no longer pursue medical school is to earn a Master's degree. As a pre-med student, your curriculum should have prepared you well to earn a Master's in Health Administration or a Master's in Public Health. These are both degrees that allow for more of a hands-off interaction in medicine than providing direct care to patients. Earning a Master's degree in one of these areas will allow you to create, implement, and maintain programs and initiatives carried out by physicians in your community. Although you may not be directly caring for patients your work in both of these fields will serve to improve lives.

Not gaining admittance into medical school can be extremely hard to deal with as most pre-medical students are high achievers and not used to failing. However, do not let your downfall lead to defeat. Although it might hurt, not gaining admittance is not the end of your dream. If you decide to reapply, there are numerous ways to strengthen your application and greatly improve your chances. If you continue to work hard and improve your application and interview skills you will gain an acceptance. Remember, a large portion of medical students do not begin immediately after undergrad and do not get discouraged if you need to reapply.

While many will choose to reapply there are some who, for numerous different reasons, will choose to not reapply. Despite not gaining admittance there are still numerous ways to positively affect people through medicine. Whether you choose to pursue a more hands-on career such as a nurse, PA, Optometrist, or work more on the administrative side, there are other options for you to make a difference without earning an MD or DO.

Conclusion

Congratulations! You have completed this book and with that, you have gained all of the knowledge needed to prepare for admission into medical school. Continue to refer back through the chapters as you progress in your journey. Perhaps taking the MCAT or interviewing at a medical school was years away when you read this book, but now, as their time approaches, the information contained has become more relevant.

While the path to medical school admittance is long and arduous, you are well on your way to success. Even though there is no secret formula to earning admission, not procrastinating and continuing to work hard are key. If you follow the strategies outlined in this book, you will have everything you need in order to create an extremely competitive application. Hopefully, you now feel more comfortable with the application process as a whole and any feelings of stress, anxiety, or being overwhelmed have been soothed.

As you move forward, remember where you came from. You were once a new college student who had very little knowledge on not only what it takes to get into medical, the specifics of the process, and everything else that is involved. Now that you are in a position of knowledge, I would encourage you to pay it forward and help those attempting to follow the same path as you. We all need help at some point in our lives and once we have improved our own situation, we often have an opportunity to give back. That is my mission for writing this book. I want to pass the knowledge and experience that I struggled to gain onto those in a similar situation as myself.

Good luck on your own journey and I wish you the most success.

Sincerely,
Ernie Morton.

For more information or to contact the author please visit:
MasteringMedicalEducation.wordpress.com

Other Books by this author: *Pre-Med, Where?*

Online Course:
*Sign up on MasteringMedicalEducation.wordpress.com